Late Diagnosed

Managing ADHD as an Adult Women

ANDREA VOSSEN

Late Diagnosed

Managing ADHD as an Adult Women

ANDREA VOSSEN

TABLE OF CONTENTS

Chapter 01
INTRODUCTION

If you are a woman who was recently diagnosed with ADHD, you may be feeling overwhelmed, confused, or relieved - but likely all 3 at the same time. On one hand, receiving a diagnosis can be a validating experience that helps explain long-standing struggles with attention, organization, and impulsivity. On the other hand, the realization that you have been living with an undiagnosed condition can be a shock to the system, potentially leading to feelings of self-doubt or regret.

Regardless of your emotional response, it is important to recognize that receiving a diagnosis is the first step towards managing your symptoms and improving your quality of life. This book is designed to provide you with practical resources, insights and strategies for managing your ADHD as an adult woman, whether you were diagnosed recently or have been living with the condition for years.

Attention-deficit/hyperactivity disorder (ADHD) is a neurodevelopmental disorder that affects an estimated 4.4% of adults in the United States and Canada. However, despite its prevalence, many adults remain undiagnosed or misdiagnosed, particularly women. In fact, research suggests that women with ADHD are often overlooked due to a variety of factors, including the tendency for girls to exhibit primarily inattentive symptoms rather than hyperactive or impulsive behaviours.

We will explore the challenges of living with ADHD as an adult woman, including common symptoms, misconceptions, and barriers to diagnosis. We will also provide guidance on developing a support system, managing time and tasks, navigating work and personal relationships, and addressing co-occurring conditions (eg. AuDHD). Our aim is to empower you to take control of your life and achieve your goals, regardless of the challenges you may face.

It is important to understand that ADHD is not a character flaw or a lack of willpower. Rather, it is a condition that affects the brain's ability to regulate attention, behavior, and emotions.

ADHD can manifest in different ways depending on the individual, and it can affect every aspect of a person's life, from academic and professional performance to personal relationships and self-esteem.

One of the challenges of living with ADHD as an adult woman is that the symptoms can be easily misunderstood or overlooked. For example, women with ADHD may struggle with disorganization, forgetfulness, and procrastination, which can be attributed to laziness or a lack of motivation. Similarly, emotional dysregulation, a common symptom of ADHD, can be mistaken for moodiness or instability.

Additionally, many women with ADHD are misdiagnosed with other conditions, such as depression or anxiety. While these conditions can co-occur with ADHD, they require different treatment approaches, and addressing them without recognizing the underlying ADHD can be ineffective or even detrimental.

Despite these challenges, it is possible to live a fulfilling life with ADHD. With the right strategies and support, individuals with ADHD can learn to manage their symptoms and thrive in their personal and professional lives. This e-book is intended to serve as a guide for adult women with ADHD who are seeking practical solutions and emotional support as they navigate the challenges of living with the condition.

In the following chapters, we will explore a variety of topics related to managing ADHD symptoms as an adult woman. Whether you are newly diagnosed or have been living with ADHD for years, we hope that this book will provide you with the tools and inspiration you need to live a fulfilling and authentic life.

Chapter 02

UNDERSTANDING ADHD SYMPTOMS

ADHD is a complex disorder that affects the brain's ability to regulate attention, behavior, and emotions. The symptoms of ADHD can manifest in different ways depending on the individual, and they can have a significant impact on daily life. In this chapter, we will explore the three core symptoms of ADHD: inattentiveness, hyperactivity, and impulsivity.

INATTENTIVENESS

One of the hallmark symptoms of ADHD is inattentiveness. Individuals with ADHD may struggle to sustain attention, focus on tasks, or follow through on commitments. This can manifest in a variety of ways, such as becoming easily distracted, losing track of time, or making careless mistakes. Inattentiveness can also lead to difficulties with organization, planning, and prioritizing tasks, which can be especially challenging in academic or professional settings.

HYPERACTIVITY

Hyperactivity is another common symptom of ADHD, although it may be more pronounced in children than in adults. Hyperactivity can manifest as restlessness, fidgeting, or excessive talking, and it may be more visible in social situations or high-energy environments. While hyperactivity may be less noticeable in adults with ADHD, they may still experience an inner sense of restlessness or difficulty sitting still.

IMPULSIVITY

Impulsivity is the third core symptom of ADHD, and it can have significant consequences for individuals with the condition. Impulsivity can manifest in impulsive decision-making, risk-taking behaviors, or difficulty controlling emotional responses. For example, individuals with ADHD may struggle to regulate their anger or frustration, leading to outbursts or conflicts with others. Impulsivity can also lead to difficulties with substance abuse, gambling, or other high-risk behaviours.

It is important to note that while inattentiveness, hyperactivity, and impulsivity are the core symptoms of ADHD, individuals with the condition may experience them in different ways and to varying degrees. For example, some individuals with ADHD may struggle primarily with inattentiveness, while others may exhibit more hyperactive or impulsive behaviors. Additionally, symptoms may be more or less pronounced depending on the context, such as in social situations versus academic or professional settings.

Understanding the symptoms of ADHD is an important step towards managing the condition. By recognizing the ways in which ADHD affects your attention, behavior, and emotions, you can begin to develop strategies for coping with the challenges that arise. In the following chapters, we will explore practical solutions for managing the symptoms of ADHD, including strategies for improving focus, regulating emotions, and developing healthy habits.

It is important to note that while medication can be an effective treatment for ADHD, it is not the only solution.

Many individuals with ADHD benefit from a combination of medication and behavioral interventions, such as therapy, coaching, or lifestyle changes. By taking a holistic approach to managing the condition, individuals with ADHD can learn to thrive in their personal and professional lives, achieving their goals and fulfilling their potential.

Chapter 03

ADHD & MEDICATION

Medication can be a highly effective tool for managing the symptoms of ADHD. While it is not a cure for the condition, medication can help to reduce the severity of symptoms, making it easier for individuals with ADHD to focus, regulate their emotions, and engage in goal-directed behavior. In this chapter, we will explore the different types of medication used to treat ADHD, their benefits and side effects, and considerations for medication management.

STIMULANT MEDICATION

Stimulant medication is the most commonly prescribed treatment for ADHD. This type of medication works by increasing the levels of certain neurotransmitters in the brain, including dopamine and norepinephrine, which play a key role in regulating attention and behavior. Stimulant medication can help to improve focus, reduce impulsivity, and increase the ability to sustain attention over time.

There are two types of stimulant medication: methylphenidate (Ritalin) and amphetamines (Adderall, Vyvanse). Methylphenidate is typically prescribed in short-acting or long-acting formulations, which can be taken multiple times a day or once a day, respectively. Amphetamines are typically prescribed in longer-acting formulations, which can be taken once a day.

While stimulant medication can be highly effective, it may not be appropriate for everyone. Stimulant medication can cause side effects such as loss of appetite, difficulty sleeping, and irritability. In rare cases, stimulant medication can also lead to more serious side effects, such as tics or cardiovascular problems. Additionally, individuals with a history of substance abuse or heart problems may not be candidates for stimulant medication.

NON-STIMULANT MEDICATION

For individuals who cannot tolerate or do not respond well to stimulant medication, there are other options available. Non-stimulant medication, such as atomoxetine (Strattera) and guanfacine (Intuniv), work by targeting different neurotransmitters in the brain, such as norepinephrine or alpha-2 receptors. These medications may be less effective than stimulants for some individuals, but they may be a good option for those who cannot take or do not respond well to stimulants.

Non-stimulant medication can also cause side effects, such as fatigue, dizziness, or stomach upset. Like stimulant medication, non-stimulant medication may not be appropriate for everyone, and it is important to discuss the risks and benefits of these medications with a healthcare provider.

MEDICATION MANAGEMENT CONSIDERATIONS
If medication is prescribed for ADHD, it is important to work closely with a healthcare provider to ensure safe and effective management. This may involve regular check-ins to monitor the individual's response to medication and adjust the dosage or formulation as needed.

It may also involve developing a plan for managing side effects or addressing concerns about medication use.

In addition to medication management, it is important to engage in other strategies for managing ADHD symptoms, such as therapy, coaching, or lifestyle changes. These interventions can help to address the underlying challenges that contribute to ADHD symptoms, such as poor time management or difficulty regulating emotions.

Medication can be a highly effective tool for managing the symptoms of ADHD. However, it is important to carefully consider the risks and benefits of medication use, and to work closely with a healthcare provider to ensure safe and effective management. In the next chapter, we will explore strategies for managing ADHD symptoms without medication, including lifestyle changes, therapy, and coaching.

Chapter 04
DEVELOPING A SUPPORT SYSTEM

If you've recently been diagnosed with ADHD as a woman, you may be feeling overwhelmed and uncertain about how to manage your symptoms. One important step you can take is to build a strong support system to help you navigate your new reality. In this chapter, we'll explore why having a support system is important for newly diagnosed women with ADHD, and provide some tips on how to develop your own.

WHY IS A SUPPORT SYSTEM SO IMPORTANT?

A support system is a group of people who provide practical and emotional support when needed. Having a support system is important for newly diagnosed women with ADHD because it can help reduce stress and anxiety, increase productivity, and improve overall well-being. The journey of managing ADHD can be difficult and isolating, and having a network of supportive individuals can provide a sense of community and validation.

Moreover, seeking help and support when needed can help you overcome the challenges of living with ADHD.

REACH OUT TO FRIENDS & FAMILY

Your loved ones can be a great source of support as you navigate life with ADHD. Talk to them about your diagnosis and how it affects you. Explain what you need from them in terms of support, whether it's practical help with household chores or emotional support. Friends and family members who are aware of your diagnosis may be better equipped to understand your behavior and offer support and assistance when you need it.

JOIN A SUPPORT GROUP

Joining a support group can provide a sense of community and validation, and help you feel less alone in your journey. There are many support groups for women with ADHD that can provide a safe space to connect with others who are going through similar experiences.

FIND A COACH

An ADHD coach can provide guidance and support in developing coping strategies and managing your symptoms. ADHD coaches are trained to help individuals with ADHD overcome the unique challenges they face, and can help you set goals and stay on track. They can also provide practical tips for managing your symptoms and improving your quality of life.

SEEK THERAPY

Therapy can be a valuable tool for managing ADHD symptoms, especially if you're struggling with anxiety or depression related to your diagnosis. A therapist can help you develop coping strategies, manage stress, and improve communication skills. It's important to find a therapist with experience working with adults with ADHD, as they will have a better understanding of your needs and challenges.

BUILD A GOOD RELATIONSHIP WITH YOUR DOCTOR

Your doctor can provide valuable guidance in managing your symptoms, including medication management and referrals to other healthcare professionals. Building a good relationship with them is important because it allows them to better understand your needs and provide the best possible care. Be open and honest about your symptoms, ask questions, and follow their advice. Your doctor can be a valuable resource in your journey of managing ADHD.

By reaching out to friends and family, joining a support group, finding an ADHD coach, seeking therapy, and building a good relationship with your doctor, you can build a strong support network to help you navigate the challenges of living with ADHD.

Remember that seeking help and support is a sign of strength, and there are people who want to support you in your journey.

Chapter 05

MINDFULNESS TECHNIQUES

Mindfulness is a practice that involves intentionally focusing on the present moment with an attitude of acceptance and non-judgment. Mindfulness techniques can be a powerful tool for managing ADHD symptoms such as inattention, impulsivity, and hyperactivity. In this chapter, we will explore mindfulness techniques and how they can be used to manage ADHD symptoms.

Mindfulness-Based Stress Reduction (MBSR)
MBSR is a program that was developed by Jon Kabat-Zinn in the 1970s to help individuals manage stress and improve well-being. MBSR involves a combination of mindfulness meditation, body awareness, and yoga. The program is typically taught over an 8-week period and includes weekly group sessions and daily home practice.

Research has shown that MBSR can be effective in reducing symptoms of ADHD. One study found that adults with ADHD who completed an 8-week MBSR program showed improvements in attention, hyperactivity, and impulsivity, as well as reductions in stress and anxiety.

MINDFUL BREATHING

Mindful breathing is a simple mindfulness technique that involves focusing on the breath and bringing attention back to the breath when the mind wanders. This technique can be particularly helpful for managing impulsivity and hyperactivity.

To practice mindful breathing, find a quiet and comfortable place to sit. Close your eyes and take a deep breath in, filling your lungs with air. Hold the breath for a few seconds, and then slowly exhale. Focus on the sensation of your breath as it enters and leaves your body. If your mind wanders, simply bring your attention back to your breath.

BODY SCAN

The body scan is a mindfulness technique that involves systematically focusing on each part of the body and noticing any sensations that are present. This technique can be helpful for managing anxiety and stress, as well as improving body awareness.

To practice the body scan, lie down in a comfortable position and close your eyes. Bring your attention to your toes and notice any sensations that are present. Slowly move your attention up through your body, noticing sensations in each part of the body. If you notice any tension or discomfort, simply observe it without judgment and continue to move through the body.

MINDFUL MOVEMENT

Mindful movement is a type of mindfulness practice that involves bringing attention to the movements of the body. This technique can be particularly helpful for managing hyperactivity and improving body awareness.

There are many different types of mindful movement practices, including yoga, tai chi, and qigong. These practices involve slow and deliberate movements that are synchronized with the breath. By focusing on the movements of the body, individuals with ADHD can improve their ability to regulate their movements, plus, reduce anxiety and impulses.

All of these techniques can be powerful tools for managing ADHD symptoms. Mindfulness-based stress reduction, mindful breathing, body scan, and mindful movement are all techniques that can be used to improve attention, reduce hyperactivity and impulsivity, and regulate emotions. By incorporating mindfulness into daily life, individuals with ADHD can develop a greater sense of awareness and improve their ability to manage their symptoms.

Chapter 06

ORGANIZATION & TIME MANAGEMENT

Individuals with ADHD often struggle with time management and task organization. These challenges can make it difficult to complete tasks, meet deadlines, and achieve goals. In this chapter, we will explore strategies for managing time and organizing tasks with ADHD.

CREATE A DAILY SCHEDULE

One of the most effective strategies for managing time and organizing tasks is to create a daily schedule. A daily schedule can help individuals with ADHD to stay focused and on-task throughout the day. To create a daily schedule, start by listing all of the tasks that need to be completed each day. Then, assign each task to a specific time slot in the schedule. Be sure to include breaks and time for self-care in the schedule. Use a planner or calendar app to keep track of the schedule.

BREAK DOWN TASKS INTO SMALLER STEPS

Another strategy for managing tasks with ADHD is to break them into smaller steps. Large tasks can be overwhelming and lead to procrastination. Breaking tasks into smaller steps can make them feel more manageable and increase the likelihood of completion.

To break tasks into smaller steps, start by identifying the overall goal of the task. Then, list all of the smaller steps that are necessary to achieve the goal. Assign a timeline to each step and use the daily schedule to plan when each step will be completed.

USE A TIMER

A timer can be a helpful tool for managing time and staying on-task. Set a timer for a specific amount of time and work on a task until the timer goes off. Take a short break, and then set the timer again for the next work session.

Using a timer can help individuals with ADHD to stay focused and avoid distractions. It can also provide a sense of structure and help with time management.

PRIORITIZE TASKS

It's important to prioritize tasks when managing time and organizing tasks with ADHD. Not all tasks are equal, and some may be more important than others.

To prioritize tasks, start by identifying which tasks are most important and which ones can wait. Focus on completing the most important tasks first, and then move on to the less important tasks. This can help individuals with ADHD to avoid feeling overwhelmed and increase their sense of accomplishment.

USE VISUAL CUES

Visual cues can be a helpful tool for managing time and organizing tasks with ADHD. Use a whiteboard, sticky notes, or a bulletin board to visually represent tasks and deadlines.

Create a visual representation of the daily schedule, including the tasks that need to be completed and the time frame for each task. Use different colors and shapes to represent different types of tasks to keep it engaging.

Time management and organizing are often very difficult for individuals with ADHD. Creating a daily schedule, breaking tasks into smaller steps, using a timer, prioritizing tasks, and using visual cues will reduce stress around time management and organizing tasks with ADHD. By incorporating these strategies into daily life, individuals with ADHD can increase their sense of control and accomplishment.

Chapter 07
EMOTIONAL REGULATION

One of the less-discussed but equally important challenges of ADHD is the difficulty in emotional regulation. Individuals with ADHD may experience intense emotions and have difficulty regulating them, leading to impulsivity, anxiety, and depression. In this chapter, we will discuss coping strategies for emotional regulation with ADHD.

PRACTICE MINDFULNESS

As previously mentioned in chapter 5, mindfulness is a technique that involves paying attention to the present moment, without judgment. Practicing mindfulness can help individuals with ADHD to become more aware of their emotions and to regulate them more effectively.

Choose a peaceful area to sit or lie down to begin practising mindfulness. Consider your breathing, focusing on the sensation of air entering and leaving your body. Bring your focus back to your breath whenever your thoughts begin to stray. Every day, spend a few minutes practising; over time, extend your practise sessions.

ENGAGE IN REGULAR EXERCISE

Exercise is a powerful tool for regulating emotions and reducing stress. Regular exercise can help individuals with ADHD to release pent-up energy and to improve their mood.

To incorporate exercise into your routine, start by finding an activity that you enjoy, such as walking, swimming, or yoga. Start with a small goal, such as walking for 10 minutes a day, and gradually increase the duration and intensity of your exercise sessions.

PRACTICE SELF-CARE

Self-care is an essential part of emotional regulation for individuals with ADHD. Taking care of yourself physically, mentally, and emotionally can help you to feel more balanced and in control. Self-care activities can include getting enough sleep, eating a healthy diet, engaging in hobbies and interests, and spending time with supportive friends and family. It's important to prioritize self-care as a regular part of your routine.

SEEK PROFESSIONAL SUPPORT

If you are struggling with emotional regulation, it can be helpful to seek professional support. A mental health professional can provide you with strategies and support for managing your emotions and regulating your mood.

There are several types of therapy that can be helpful for individuals with ADHD, including cognitive-behavioral therapy, dialectical behavior therapy, and mindfulness-based therapy. Medication may also be an option, depending on your individual needs and preferences.

CREATE A SUPPORTIVE ENVIRONMENT

Creating a supportive environment can also be helpful for emotional regulation with ADHD. Surround yourself with people who understand and support you, and who can offer you encouragement and validation.
It's also important to create a physical environment that is conducive to emotional regulation. Minimize distractions and clutter, and create a space that feels calm and relaxing.

Emotional regulation can be a significant challenge for individuals with ADHD. Coping strategies such as mindfulness, regular exercise, self-care, seeking professional support, and creating a supportive environment can all be helpful in regulating emotions and improving mood. By incorporating these strategies into your routine, you can increase your sense of emotional control and well-being.

Chapter 08
MANAGING WORKLIFE

Managing ADHD in the workplace can be a challenge. The fast-paced, high-stress environment can exacerbate symptoms such as distractibility, impulsivity, and difficulty with time management. In this chapter, we will discuss some tips for managing ADHD in the workplace. Many techniques previously discussed in chapter 6 can also be applied to improving your work life and work-life balance.

STRUCTURED ROUTINE

Establishing a routine can be incredibly helpful for individuals with ADHD. Creating a consistent schedule for tasks such as checking emails, attending meetings, and completing projects can help you to stay on track and manage your time more effectively.

BREAK DOWN LARGE TASKS

Breaking down larger tasks into smaller, more manageable steps can make them feel less overwhelming. This approach can also help you to focus on one task at a time, reducing the likelihood of distraction and procrastination.

USE VISUAL AIDS

Visual aids such as calendars, to-do lists, and sticky notes can help individuals with ADHD to stay organized and on-task. Consider using color-coding or highlighting techniques to help important information stand out.

TAKE BREAKS

Taking regular breaks can help to reduce stress and fatigue, allowing you to focus more effectively when you return to work. Try to incorporate short breaks into your schedule, such as taking a walk around the office or stretching at your desk.

MINIMIZE DISTRACTIONS

Distractions can be a significant challenge for individuals with ADHD in the workplace. Try to minimize distractions by finding a quiet place to work, using noise-cancelling headphones, or using website blockers to limit your access to social media or other distracting websites.

PRIORITIZE SELF-CARE

Self-care is essential for managing ADHD in the workplace. Prioritizing healthy habits such as exercise, healthy eating, and getting enough sleep can help to reduce stress and improve focus and productivity.

COMMUNICATE WITH YOUR EMPLOYER

It can be helpful to communicate with your employer about your ADHD and any accommodations you may need to perform your job effectively. This can include things such as flexible work hours, a quiet workspace, or access to technology or tools that can help you to manage your symptoms.

SEEK PROFESSIONAL SUPPORT

If you are struggling to manage your ADHD in

the workplace, it can be helpful to seek professional support. A mental health professional can provide you with strategies and support for managing your symptoms and improving your job performance.

In summary, managing ADHD in the workplace can be a challenge, but it's not impossible. By creating a structured routine, breaking down tasks into smaller steps, using visual aids, taking breaks, minimizing distractions, prioritizing self-care, communicating with your employer, and seeking professional support, you can effectively manage your symptoms and perform your job more effectively.

Remember to be patient and compassionate with yourself, and to celebrate your successes along the way.

Chapter 09

OVERCOMING SHAME & STIGMA

Getting diagnosed with ADHD as a woman can be a life-changing experience. It can provide clarity and understanding for a lifetime of challenges, and give you access to effective treatments and resources. However, it's not uncommon for women who are diagnosed later in life to experience feelings of shame and stigma surrounding their diagnosis. In this chapter, we'll explore how to overcome these negative feelings and embrace your new reality with positivity and self-compassion.

UNDERSTANDING SHAME & STIGMA

Shame is a negative emotion that can arise when we feel that we have fallen short of our expectations or the expectations of others. It can lead to feelings of worthlessness, inadequacy, and isolation. Stigma is the negative attitudes and beliefs that others hold towards individuals with a particular condition or trait.

Both shame and stigma can be significant barriers to seeking help and support, and can make it difficult to move forward after receiving an ADHD diagnosis.

PRACTICE SELF-COMPASSION

Self-compassion involves treating ourselves with the same kindness, concern, and support that we would offer to a good friend. It involves recognizing that we are not alone in our struggles and accepting ourselves, flaws and all. Instead of focusing on the negative aspects of ADHD, try to focus on the positive qualities that it can bring, such as creativity, spontaneity, and hyper-focus. Remember that ADHD is a medical condition, not a personal failing, and that you deserve the same love and respect as anyone else.

CONNECT WITH OTHERS

Connecting with others who share your experiences can be a powerful way to overcome shame and stigma.

Joining a support group or seeking out other women with ADHD can provide a sense of community and validation. Sharing your experiences and hearing from others who have gone through similar struggles can help you feel less alone and more understood. There are many online communities and social media groups that can connect you with other women with ADHD, and there are also in-person support groups available in many areas.

EDUCATE YOURSELF & OTHERS

Educating yourself about ADHD can help you understand your diagnosis and overcome negative stereotypes and beliefs. Learn about the science behind ADHD and the effective treatments that are available. Share what you learn with others in your life, including family members, friends, and coworkers. You may be surprised at the level of understanding and support you receive when you approach the topic in an open and informative manner.

SEEK PROFESIONAL HELP

If feelings of shame and stigma are interfering with your ability to manage your ADHD symptoms or move forward with your life, seeking professional help can be an effective way to overcome them. A therapist or counselor who is familiar with ADHD can provide support and guidance in managing these feelings and developing coping strategies. They can also help you develop self-esteem and confidence in your abilities, and provide a safe and supportive space to explore your emotions and experiences.

CELEBRATE YOUR SUCCESSES

Finally, it's important to celebrate your successes, no matter how small they may seem. ADHD can present many challenges, but it can also bring many strengths and unique perspectives. Celebrate your ability to manage your symptoms, your successes in your personal and professional life, and your ability to navigate the world in your own unique way. Remember that ADHD is a part of who you are, but it doesn't define you. You are a whole and complex person, with many strengths and abilities to offer the world.

Receiving a late ADHD diagnosis as a woman can be a challenging experience, but it doesn't have to be a negative one. By practicing self-compassion, connecting with others, educating yourself and others, seeking professional help, and celebrating your successes, you can overcome feelings

Chapter 10
MOVING FORWARD

After receiving diagnosis, it may feel like your entire life has been turned upside down, but it is essential to remember that ADHD is just a part of who you are, and it doesn't define you. Instead, it is an opportunity to gain a better understanding of yourself and learn how to navigate your life with a new set of tools. In the following chapter, we summarize the tools and resources previously discussed in this book in more detail to encourage a stronger understanding of your relationship with ADHD.

One way to move forward is to embrace your personal strengths and talents. People with ADHD often possess unique abilities and strengths, such as creativity, out-of-the-box thinking, and hyperfocus. Focusing on these strengths can help you to build self-confidence and improve your self-image. Identifying your strengths can also help you to create strategies that take advantage of these strengths while minimizing the impact of your ADHD symptoms.

Developing a positive outlook is critical in moving forward after an ADHD diagnosis. It is essential to recognize that ADHD is a medical condition, and it is not your fault that you have it. Instead of dwelling on the negative aspects of ADHD, it's important to focus on the positive aspects and think about how your ADHD can be an asset. With a positive outlook, you can tackle challenges head-on and take pride in your achievements.

Setting and achieving goals is another important aspect of moving forward after an ADHD diagnosis. Goal setting can help you stay focused and motivated, and it can give you a sense of purpose. When setting goals, it's important to make them specific, measurable, and achievable. You may want to break larger goals into smaller, more manageable steps, and celebrate each small achievement along the way.

Building a Support System is essential in managing ADHD symptoms and achieving success. Having a supportive network of friends, family, and professionals can make a significant difference in your life. Seek out people who are understanding and accepting of your diagnosis and can provide you with emotional support and practical guidance.

In addition to building a support system, it is also important to seek out professional help. Many healthcare professionals specialize in helping adults with ADHD, and they can provide you with the tools and resources you need to manage your symptoms effectively. With the help of a professional, you can develop a personalized plan that addresses your specific needs and goals.

Late ADHD diagnosis as a female can be a difficult experience, but it can also be incredibly rewarding in growth and self-discovery. By embracing your personal strengths and talents, developing a positive outlook, and setting achievable goals, you can navigate your life with greater confidence and success.

Remember that you are not alone and that there are many resources available to help you manage your symptoms and achieve your goals.